How Large Things Get Completed :

THE AstonISHING ELEMENTS THAT IMPEND EVERY PROJECT'S SUCCESS.

By

Joseph F. Crawford

Copyright © by Joseph F. Crawford 2024. All rights reserved. Before this document is duplicated or reproduced in any manner, the publisher's consent must be gained. Therefore, the contents within can neither be stored electronically, transferred, nor kept in a database. Neither in Part nor full can the document be copied, scanned, faxed, or retained without approval from the publisher or creator.

TABLE OF CONTENTS

Introduction

How can a vision evolve into a strategy that brings about a victorious new reality? I'll tell you a story now. If you depart from California in particular, you might have heard about it.

In 2008, voters in the Golden State were asked to picture themselves riding on a modern, silver train at Union Station in downtown Los Angeles. As it leaves the station, the train moves silently through the unending gridlock and urban sprawl before picking up speed and exploding into the Central Valley's vast open areas, passing through the countryside in a blur. It's breakfast time. The train slows and glides into another station by the time waiters empty coffee cups and plates. This is San Francisco's downtown. The entire journey took two and a half hours, which is not much more than the typical Los Angeles resident would need to drive to the airport, go through security, board a plane, and wait in line for takeoff on the tarmac. The train ticket was $86 in price. The California High-Speed Rail project was named for it. It would link Silicon Valley, the world's center of technology, with two of the greatest cities on earth The center of advanced technologies worldwide. Although the term "visionary" is overused, this truly was visionary. And by 2020 it would be operational at a total cost of $33 billion.2. Voters in a state-wide referendum approved. Work got underway. It has been fourteen years as of this writing. There are still many unanswered questions regarding the project, but one thing is for certain: it won't turn out to be the fairy tale that was anticipated. Following voter approval of the proposal, building got underway at a few locations along the route, but frequent delays plagued the project. Plans were modified time and again. Estimates of costs shot up to $43 billion, $68 billion, $77 billion, and eventually over $83 billion. Right now, as I write, the highest estimate is 1 Educating note: In this and other places in the story, "me" and "I" refer to Bent Flyvbjerg. 2 A variety of scenarios were given for the estimated cost of the tickets, ranging from $68 to $104. The project was expected to cost between $32.785 billion and $33.625 billion in

total. The California High-Speed Rail
Authority's Financial Plan from 1999
can be viewed here. Similarly, the
California High-Speed Rail Authority's
Business Plan for the California High-
Speed Train from 2008 can be viewed
here.

The 21st-century Safe and Reliable
High-Speed Passenger Train Bond Act
was passed by the California High-Speed
Rail Authority in 2008. AB-3034. 3.
California High-Speed Rail Authority
(2012), Building California's Future: A
Revised Business Plan for the California
High-Speed Rail Program, The 2014
Connecting California Business Plan was
published by the California High-Speed
Rail Authority in Sacramento, California.
The California High-Speed Rail
Authority (2016) published a business
plan titled "Connecting and
Transforming California" in Sacramento,
California. California High-Speed Rail

Authority, Sacramento, California (2018), 2018.

4 The governor of California declared in 2019 that the state would only finish a 171-mile stretch of the route—between the towns of Merced and Bakersfield in the Central Valley—at an estimated cost of over $23 billion. But the project will come to an end once the inland stretch is finished. A later governor will have to determine whether to restart the project and, if so, how to raise the approximately $80 billion (or whatever amount would be needed by then) needed to expand the rails and link Los Angeles and San Francisco.

.4 To put things in perspective, the cost of the Merced to Bakersfield line alone is equal to or greater than the gross domestic output of Iceland, Honduras, and over a hundred other nations combined. And between two cities that most people outside of California have never heard of, that money will be used to build the most advanced train route in North America. It will be the "bullet train to nowhere," as detractors have described it. How can ideas turn into plans that result in accomplished projects? not in this manner. A lofty goal is a beautiful thing. California was audacious. It had lofty dreams. But a vision alone is insufficient, even with mountains of cash. I'll tell you one more tale. Although this one is unclear, I believe it brings us closer to the answers we need. Danish government authorities had an idea in the early 1990s. Denmark is a small nation, home to fewer people than New York City, but it is wealthy, generous with its international aid, and committed to seeing its money used for good. Education is one of the best things there is. Together with colleagues from other governments, the Danish officials decided to provide funding for Nepal's

education system, which is located in the Himalayas. Twenty thousand classrooms and schools would be constructed, most of them in the most isolated and impoverished areas. In 1992, work would start. Twenty years would pass.5.
 The background of international aid is Strewn with boogers, and this project might have made matters worse. Even so, it was completed in 2004 within budget, with eight business plans, California High-Speed Rail Authority, Sacramento, California; California High-Speed Rail Authority (2021), 2020 Recovery and Transformation Business Plan, The 2020 Business Plan Ridership & Revenue Forecasting Report was released by the California High-Speed Rail Authority in Sacramento, California. The Revised Draft 2020 Business Plan Capital Cost Basis of Estimate Report was also released by the California High-Speed Rail Authority in Sacramento,

California. 4 High-Speed Rail Authority of California (2021). California High-Speed Rail Authority, Revised Draft 2020 Business Plan Capital Cost Basis of Estimate Report, CA.
5. See Bent Flyvbjerg, "Four Ways To Scale Up: Smart, Dumb, Forced, and Fumbled," Said Business School Working Papers, Oxford University, 2021, for a detailed description of the Nepal school project.

Five years ahead of schedule. Following this, there was a nationwide increase in education levels, which had several beneficial effects, chief among them being an increase in the proportion of female students enrolled in school. Even so, the schools managed to survive: Almost 9,000 people perished in the 2015 Nepal earthquake, many of them were crushed to death in crumbling houses. But first, the schools were built to withstand earthquakes. They were on their feet. The Bill and Melinda Gates Foundation now utilizes the initiative as a model for how to increase school attendance, especially for females, to enhance health. Six On that project, I served as the planner.7. Although I was happy with the outcome at the time, I didn't give it much thought. Since it was my first major project, 'e simply accomplished what we stated we would do, which was to transform a vision into a plan that was completed on schedule. I am an academic as well as a planner, and the more I researched how large projects succeed or fail, the more I realized that my experience in Nepal was unusual. It was anything but normal, in fact. The data will demonstrate that large-scale undertakings that fulfill their promises are uncommon. Normal has a lot more California High-Speed Rail-like aesthetics. I would later generalize my conclusions regarding megaproject management to say that "average practice is a disaster, best practice is an outlier."8 Why do large initiatives have such a poor track record? More crucially, though, what about the seldom but alluring exceptions? When so many others fail, why do they succeed? If we simply had good fortune delivering the schools in Nepal? Or might we try it once more?   I've spent years responding to similar inquiries as a planning and management professor. I've been applying my solutions for many years as a consultant. I'll put them into print in this book.   Six Models for International Health, 2022. "What Action Did Nepal Take?" Retrieved April 6, 2022, from 7. The project is called the Basic and Primary Education Program, or simply BPEP. Hans Laurits Jørgensen, a Danish architect, and I collaborated to design prototype classrooms and schools.

The project was designed and programmed by me. Subsequently, the schools were built over the course of 12 years by a delivery crew. Though much as I loved being involved in the day-to-day planning and execution of projects, I had determined that my major vocation would be as a university professor, so I politely declined the offer to lead the delivery team. In-depth academic research would be necessary, in my opinion, to fully comprehend the fundamental causes of what makes projects function. I therefore went back to Denmark and my professorship to complete the study, initially at University and then at Delft University. The University of Oxford in the United Kingdom, the University of Technology in the Netherlands, the IT University of Copenhagen in Denmark, the University of Oxford in the United Kingdom, and the University of Technology in The

Netherlands. 8 Bent Flyvbjerg, ed., The Oxford Handbook of Megaproject Management (Oxford: Oxford University Press), pp. 1–18. Flyvbjerg, Bent, 2017, "Introduction: The Iron Law of Megaproject Management."

Megaprojects, or extremely large projects, are the center of my work, and there are many distinctive aspects to that field. For example, navigating national politics and international bond markets is not something that the typical home remodeler has to deal with.

But that is a topic for another book. The universal drivers of the project's success and failure are what I'm interested in here. That clarifies the title. Big Things is an acknowledgment of my proficiency in megaprojects, which are enormous by any measure. However, "big" varies. Remodeling a home can easily rank among the most costly, difficult, and complex projects that the average homeowner has ever taken on. For them, getting it right is just as important as for governments and companies to determine the outcome of megaprojects. It truly is a "big thing." What then are the common factors that distinguish successful people from unsuccessful ones?

Power and Psychology

Psychology is one. People think, judge, and make decisions in any large project, which is defined by those in charge as a project that is large, complex, ambitious, and dangerous. Psychology is also at work when thinking, judging, and making judgments; this is seen, for example, when optimism is present. Power is another. In any large undertaking, individuals and groups vie for resources and positions. Power exists where rivalry and backstabbing exist. For example, a politician or CEO pushing through a pet project. Projects of all sizes, from kitchen makeovers to skyscrapers, are driven by psychology and power. They can be found in projects using bits and bytes, bricks and mortar, or any other kind of material. They can be found anywhere there is an enthusiastic individual who wants to take a vision and turn it into a plan that will make it a reality. It could be anything from adding another gem to the Manhattan skyline to starting a new company, traveling to Mars, creating a new product, altering an organization, creating a program, organizing a conference, writing a book, organizing a family wedding, or remodeling and completely changing a house.   It is reasonable to anticipate that initiatives of all stripes will follow certain patterns when universal drivers are at work. Additionally, there are. The most typical is nicely depicted via the bullet train to nowhere in California. With great anticipation, the proposal was authorized and development got underway. But issues quickly spread. Development stalled. There were more issues. Things continued to slow down. The project took forever. I'll explain why I refer to this pattern as "think fast, act slow" later. It is a telltale sign of failed endeavors.

 Contrarily, successful initiatives typically follow the opposite pattern and move fast toward completion. That was the course of the Nepal schools initiative. Similarly, the Hoover Dam was completed two years ahead of time and somewhat under budget in less than five years.9. The first of the famous Boeing 747s took 28 months to develop and manufacture by Boeing.10 In late January 2001, Apple hired its first employee to begin the development of what would become the iconic iPod. In March of the same year, the project received official approval, and in

November of that same year, the first iPod was distributed to customers.11 Between October 2004 and February 2005, Amazon Prime, the retailer's wildly popular membership and free shipping program, evolved from a nebulous concept to a public announcement.12 In a matter of weeks, the first SMS texting application was created.

 I inquired as to how a plan is developed from a vision to create a victorious new reality. That is the response, as we shall see: Consider carefully and quickly.

Chapter 1

Act Quickly, Think Slowly

.

The cornerstone of successful business execution, which is inherently innovative, intricate, and hazardous, is projects, programs, and portfolios. Every project has a different set of goals, stakeholders, and resources, which means that getting from the existing situation (the project start) to the intended state (the project outcomes) can be a difficult and uncertain journey. The optimal route is only discovered after a journey filled with occasionally traumatic encounters that illuminate the way. The "best path" for business execution is unknown, and this uncertainty plays a major role in project failure. Furthermore, in order to address this uncertainty, conventional risk management techniques have proven to be inadequate. Risk and uncertainty, even less so in the current rapidly evolving technological and economic landscape. The results of a study of

250,000 initiatives, which showed that 72% of them were judged as either "failed" or insufficient in their original goals, lend credence to this point of view (Standish, 2001). Projects must be managed and carried out in a way that takes into account the complexity of their settings if they are to be more successful (Fawford & Ward, 2006). Projects ought to be carried out quickly and nimbly so they can adjust to changing circumstances. And to achieve this, a fundamental change in the methods for identifying, evaluating, and managing risk is required.

Consider Slowly

Project planning and control have been the main focuses of traditional approaches to risk management (Atkinson, et al., 2006). While meticulous planning should not be undervalued, many projects are too complicated to be fully addressed to and project planning, particularly in the unveiling technology era. As a result, in order to handle the actual execution of projects, flexibility and agility become essential qualities (Huchzermeier & Loch, 2001). Flexibility is the capacity to respond to change, while agility is the pace at which one responds to change, according to Gong and Janssen (2012). Conversely, uncertainty has frequently been described only as "the unknown" (Stewart & Fortune, 1995). The problem is in the fact that people tend to rely primarily on information that confirms prior experiences, even in situations where we have access to the required knowledge to learn what we don't know. According to Kahneman, Lovallo, and Sibony (2011), this means that when faced with risk and uncertainty during project execution, project managers and their teams unconsciously rely primarily on the evidence that supports the initial project plan, endangering the success of the project. This way of thinking and making decisions is referred to as "System 1 thinking" by Kahneman (2011).Because System 1 thinking is rapid, simple, and intuitive, it frequently results in poor conclusions that are based on pre-implementation preparation. So, identifying, evaluating, and managing risks using System 1 thinking may lead to less adaptable and agile project execution. On the other hand, System 2 thinking, sometimes referred to as slow thinking, is deliberate, controlled, and labor-intensive (Kahneman, 2011). By approaching project risk and uncertainty "slowly," one can identify and analyze risk more accurately and manage it more nimbly as the project is being carried out (Shleifer, 2012).

Move Quickly

Stewart and Fortune (1995), in their well-known work on systems thinking and risk in IT projects, examined the risk stages related to the project life cycle. They recognized risk assessment and identification only at the feasibility and analysis stages of the project lifecycle. However, this perspective is constraining when new and unexpected risks emerge during implementation. Events that do not conform to the original project plan, such as design or specification changes, often create uncertainty and panic that in turn lead to quick decision-making and action-taking without fully considering the broader implications (Atkinson al., 2006). For example, the consequences of scheduling, supplier deadlines, or even communication channels can impact various stakeholders, and ultimately the success of the project. Thinking fast, or System 1 thinking, produces flawed decisions about implementation stage risk. However, when System 1 and System 2 thinking are mixed, a natural synergy is created that allows for flexibility and agility by slowing down when analysis and planning require focus and speeding up when action is needed. System 2 thinking must be applied during the risk identification and assessment stages, when a comprehensive study is necessary, for this strategy to be effective. However, the comprehensive analysis allows for quicker measures to neutralize threats or take advantage of opportunities when risks materialize and a swift response is needed, either to carry out the pre-planned contingency plans or to react to the evolving nature of risks. Consequently, given the rate of change and technology The way we think about risk at the project execution stage must thus adjust to a slower thinking style mixed with faster actions due to the rapid pace of change and technological innovation. Slower thinking will enable project teams to identify, evaluate, and manage risk more accurately and purposefully. Project teams will then have the flexibility they need to manage risk and uncertainty efficiently and effectively as a result.

Large-scale project performance is considerably poorer than it appears.

The pace at which large initiatives fail is startling. These projects take months or even years to complete and involve massive resource consumption, whether they be post merger integrations, new growth strategies, or big technology installs. However, numerous studies have demonstrated, they frequently produce dismal returns—well over half the time, according to some estimates. Furthermore, their costs go beyond money. When this happens, workers who have put in a lot of effort to finish their portion of the task become discouraged. "I've been on dozens of task teams in my career, and I've never actually seen one that produced a result," a middle management at a major pharmaceutical business told us.

The issue is that project teams using the traditional method of project management become more focused on creating recommendations, new technologies, and partial solutions than they are on the final product. Naturally, the idea is to combine these into a design that will enable the completion of the project, but when a project involves When a large number of people are working for extended periods of time, it can be challenging for managers to anticipate all the activities and work streams that will be required. Certain aspects are nearly always left off the plan, especially in highly specialized engineering projects like manufacturing an airplane, unless the final outcome is clearly known. Furthermore, even if all the necessary tasks have been planned, it could be difficult or even impossible to tie them all together once they are finished.

Project managers employ budgets, schedules, and plans to lower the risk of improper execution of assigned tasks, or what is known as "execution risk." They invariably overlook these two additional crucial risks: the "integration risk," which states that the various activities won't come together in the end, and the "white space risk," which states that some necessary activities won't be identified in advance, creating gaps in the project plan. Therefore, even if project teams complete their work perfectly, on schedule, and within budget, the project as a whole could not produce the desired outcomes.

Over the course of the last 20 years, we have worked with hundreds of teams, and we have discovered that managers may decrease the possibility that important tasks will be omitted from the plan and raise the likelihood that everything will be correctly integrated in the end by approaching the design of complicated projects in a new way. The secret is to add to the overall Create a number of mini projects, or what we refer to as rapid-results initiatives. Each one will be staffed with a team that will be in charge of a smaller version of the desired overall result, and they will all be able to produce their results rapidly.

Let's examine the potential impact of that. Let's take an example where your objective is to equip your sales force with a customer relationship management (CRM) system in order to double sales revenue within a two-year period. Using a standard project management methodology, you may assign tasks to different teams, such as researching and installing software, analyzing the many client interactions the company has (email, phone, in-person, etc.), developing training programs, and so on. However, when you begin implementing the program many months later, you may find that the Salespeople don't see the advantages. Thus, they decline even if they might be able to input the necessary data into the system. Indeed, a number of CRM initiatives at significant companies have failed because of this very issue but imagine how things may go if the project included some initiatives aimed at getting results quickly. Within four months, one team might be tasked with increasing the revenues of a small number of users—let's say, one sales group in one region—by 25%. Team members would presumably use all of the previously mentioned actions, but in order to achieve their objective—which is a microcosm of the larger objective—they would need to determine what, if anything, is still missing from their current plans as they move forward. As they traveled, they would, for instance, if they were to uncover the salespeople's resistance, they would be forced to inform the sales team of the advantages of the system. The group may also find that there are additional problems that need to be resolved, like how to split commissions on sales that come from collaborative or cross-selling initiatives. Their effort would then serve as a model for the following teams, who would either take part in other rapid-results projects or implement the system across the entire company once all the bugs have been worked out on a modest scale. but this time with more assurance that the project will have the desired effect on

sales income. The team would feel good about providing genuine value, the corporation would see an early return on its investment, and it would learn new things from the team's work.
We'll examine rapid-results initiatives in detail in the pages that follow, utilizing case studies to demonstrate how college projects are chosen, planned, and managed in tandem with more conventional project operations.

Chapter2

The Commitment Fallacy:

Why do people stick to their beliefs even when contradicted by evidence? What is the Fallacy of Commitment? The escalation of commitment, or commitment fallacy, refers to our propensity to stick with our previous behaviors—especially those that we have publicly demonstrated—even when they do not yield the desired results. Consider yourself nearing the end of your first year of college , concentrating on cell biology and anatomy. Nobody was surprised that you decided to pursue a career in medicine as this was always your dream to attend medical school and become a doctor. You signed up for an elective course on the history of modern Europe during your first semester. Even though you didn't particularly enjoy your foundational anatomy studies, you discovered that you were engrossed in the history elective you had chosen on a whim. You took a number of other history classes in your second semester and devoted your leisure time studying the topics covered in class because you found it to be so enjoyable. There has been a persistent voice in the back of your mind encouraging you to switch to history as your major and earn a Bachelor of Arts throughout the entire academic year. But this choice contradicts everything you've ever expressed about yourself and your long-term objectives. While it's acceptable to have second thoughts, you may feel under pressure to maintain consistency. Despite the fact that changing your major is what you really want to accomplish, you are hesitant to do so because of the commitment fallacy. Making wise selections is seriously hampered by the belief that our actions now and in the future must conform to our prior words and deeds. This is particularly true in cases where our previous decisions have had bad effects. It can also be difficult when our previous actions conflict with our principles now. Refusing to modify one's position might hinder personal development in addition to producing bad outcomes. It is highly adaptive to be able to see the shortcomings in our previous actions and use those lessons to improve. In the end, it will give us more self-awareness and enable us to make more thoughtful, rational judgments. systemic impacts The commitment fallacy is a problem that can get worse when someone in a position of authority demonstrates it. There have been suggestions that this happens in companies where the decision-maker is doubting their position. Within the societal structure. Additionally, according to researchers, this conduct is typical when someone in charge of establishing policy is "anxious about [their] standing among [constituents" when ideas are being proposed.1. This is concerning since commitment fallacy can lead to poor decision-making, and these decisions are frequently crucial ones.

How it impacts the product

The commitment fallacy is very common while developing new products. Even when a product's cost outweighs its value, people who take on leadership roles early in the pipeline are less likely to give up on it, according to research by Jeffrey B. Schmidt and Roger J. Calantone. Furthermore, compared to individuals who assume leadership roles later in the product development process, people who start the project are less likely to witness its failures.[11] It's crucial to keep going in order to prevent this to get feedback when a product is developed. A diverse viewpoint can be obtained by adding more "on the outside" team members later on, which can help the business save time, money, and resources. The promotion of open-mindedness is crucial. This entails fostering an atmosphere where individuals are at ease enough to generate fresh concepts and take into account other viewpoints. It's also critical to promote with cooperation and the idea that creative solutions can be achieved by teamwork.

Chapter 3 :

From Right To Left Thinking

The idea of thinking from the right to the left has received a lot of attention lately. The idea centers on the capacity to think creatively, to weigh all aspects of a problem, and to approach problems from several angles. Success in business and innovation has been demonstrated to greatly benefit from this way of thinking since it fosters the creation of fresh concepts and tactics that can be applied to promote an organization's goals. Businesses can see beyond the conventional methods of doing things and create novel solutions that can provide them a competitive edge by adopting a right-to-left strategy. An outline of right-to-left thinking will be given in this piece, along with a discussion of its advantages and offer some advice on how to realize its full creative and commercial potential.

Right-to-Left Thinking: What Is It?

Thinking from right to left involves examining an issue from all angles, weighing all potential solutions, and selecting the best one. It entails taking a fresh approach to the issue rather than concentrating just on the conventional methods. It's a kind of creative thinking that pushes people to consider options other than the traditional ones while addressing issues. This way of thinking is advantageous because it enables companies to create solutions that are distinctive and provide them a competitive edge.

The benefits of right to left thinking

Thinking from the right to the left provides many advantages for the success of a company and innovation. First of all, it enables companies to approach issue resolution in a more inventive manner. It has been said that this kind of thinking pushes people to think beyond the box and to investigate solutions they may not have entertained before. This may spark the creation of cutting-edge tactics that offer benefits over competitor

Second, firms are able to make better decisions when they apply right to left thinking. Businesses that use a right-to-left perspective are able to weigh all relevant information before making a choice. This guarantees that companies take the greatest option for their company.

Thirdly, companies can learn more about their clients by applying right-to-left thinking. Businesses can better understand the requirements and desires of their customers by approaching problems from many angles, and they can then create solutions that address those demands.

Lastly, it can support companies in being more flexible and adaptable. Companies are able to create solutions that provide them a competitive edge and quickly adjust to changes in the market.

How to Unlock Your Left-to-Right Thinking

To fully realize the potential of right-to-left thinking in business and innovation, there are a few strategies to try.

It's critical to keep the customer in mind. Businesses may create solutions that satisfy customers' needs and give them a competitive edge by learning about their needs and wants.

Ensuring that all members of the organization participate in the decision-making process is crucial. This guarantees that while making judgments, all points of view are taken into account. It's critical to provide team members with enough time to generate fresh concepts and brainstorm.

Giving input on concepts and solutions is crucial. Team members can improve their ideas and solutions as a result thinking creatively from the right to the left provides several advantages for the success of the company and innovation. It enables companies to adopt a more inventive strategy to problem-solving, improve their decision-making, learn more about their clients, and become more adaptable and change-responsive. Encouraging people to think creatively and from a variety of angles, keeping the customer in mind, including everyone in the decision-making process, giving team members time to develop new ideas and brainstorm, and offering feedback on concepts and solutions are all crucial to maximizing the potential of right-to-left thinking. Businesses that adopt a right-to-left strategy might create novel solutions that provide them a competitive edge.

Begin with the most fundamental query of all: "Why."

In order for companies to learn about and comprehend the society and economy they operate in, they must ask themselves "why." Despite its significance, it is evident that different organizations follow different paths when it comes to asking why, as many of them do not employ the same strategy. In business, the inquiries that are asked most frequently center around the "what," "where," "when," or "how."

Maybe there is a personality type that manifests itself in professionals that ask these kinds of "big picture" questions and inquiries aimed at greater discoveries. It's also possible that more individuals might think about asking more of these kinds of inquiries, but they might be pressed for time and believe that by getting to the point quickly, they'll save time.

Determining the Significance of Declarations

So why not inquire as to why? The short answer is that there's a reason "why" queries are helpful. Before delving further into the specifics, experts in the product development field, for instance, may discover that asking themselves why they are doing something is a useful way to foster knowledge. As a result of their connections within a larger framework, the details become easier to comprehend and recall.

Think about a theater play or movie as an example. Does reading the story help you recall the characters more than just looking at the array of characters? It is preferable to examine the cast's characteristics and specifics through a story rather than a comprehensive reference list. Thus, the link between the subject matter and our sense of significance is constructed by the context of what is being taught.

The Value of "Why" in Analytical Thought

"Why" inquiries are the ones that make you take a step back and use more critical thinking skills. Do you occasionally become so engrossed in the minutiae that you create a project plan that diverges from the original objective? Having worked with both huge enterprises and the government, I have witnessed the typical project problem of creeping scope on multiple occasions.

When more general goals and objectives are misinterpreted, what good is it to concentrate on particular details? Is there a legitimate reason to keep doing something if the person is unable to explain why they are doing it? Not responding to the simplest of queries imply that they ought to put more effort into learning before acting. The next time you have to make a decision, consider the circumstances and ask yourself why you chose what you did. Consider how to engage a client or customer at a higher level during your initial meeting, where it will be easier to find answers to ongoing problems or uncover new prospects. What makes them require help? Put that first and foremost if you want to boost participation and hasten company success. Bring your efforts back to the main objective whenever you become distracted by anything else than the "why." The motivation behind an action should not be secondary; rather, it should be the primary motivator.

Keep in mind that accountability comes together with the enormous power of "why"! Since everyone has a unique communication style, asking certain people too many "why" inquiries may make it difficult for them to concentrate and complete tasks. Recognize the authority and motivation behind your actions, and know when to seek clarification. This could lead to more fruitful discussions and interactions as well as time and energy savings.

How Your Funding Plan Can Benefit From Asking Why?

Asking "Why?" is important for organizations in all aspects, but it's particularly important when deciding where to spend in company planning throughout the fiscal year and when organizing business activities. It is crucial to think about what your company wants to accomplish this year and "Why" we want to accomplish these goals when making plans for the future. A company can arrange its finances after determining the purpose of the project it is working on this year. For instance, a manufacturing company would know where to search for funding if its "Why" is to "improve total daily productivity outputs" and it wants to undertake a capital and technology adoption project. The company now realizes that in order to accomplish its "why," it will require new machinery, equipment, and employee training to run it. This can help the company develop a financial plan by utilizing government funding opportunities, more information about which can be found on the Navigating the Government financial Process Slide Deck.

"Why" fosters our development

Ask yourself why you are where you are in life and why you want to change if you ever feel trapped or wonder where it's heading. To transform your life, it's critical to ask yourself questions. We can better grasp how and where we wish to go in life by asking ourselves "why." More broadly, the question "why" has the power to change our lives and the lives of all people. It assists us in bringing about the desired change.

"Why" aids in our comprehension of a goal.

Have we ever wondered "why" kids study the material that is taught to them? Does what we studied in school still have any relevance to our lives now, and if so, why? We have the opportunity to transform education to make it more relevant and assist our kids in understanding the goal of their education by asking "why."

"Why" promotes sincerity.

Asking "why" enables us to face our anxieties and provide a sincere explanation for our feelings. Asking "why" can help create honest communication channels that strengthen bonds between people. It offers us the ability to reflect on and challenge our presumptions. It assists us in discovering who we are, whether the decisions and opinions we have are truly our own, and what we genuinely stand for. Asking "why" opens the door to a mind-blowing, life-changing encounter.

Chapter 4:

Do You Have Any Experience?

Technology and digital technologies have completely changed how businesses compete, run, and market their goods and services. Many have therefore declared that experience is no longer a company's main selling point—rather, it is now its talent. The idea appears to have increased as consumers' access to information online has increased and their perception of the value of experience has decreased.

Rethink your thoughts.

Although the world has evolved, human needs have not altered. Consumers still want to feel confident that the companies they do business with are reliable, superior, and attentive to their demands. Put another way, experience counts whether it is gained in person or virtually. Businesses need to realize that customers purchase more than simply goods or services. Businesses ought to understand that People frequently purchase products based on their self-perception. Additionally, businesses must go above and above to make customers feel valued in inflationary times.

What does experience mean in the business world?

Experience is a crucial component of any enterprise. The way this reality is currently presented has changed, but the fact itself has not altered with the times. Ten years ago, prospective buyers went to a car dealership or a vacation agency to gather information and decide what to buy. Nowadays, a growing number of consumers conduct online research before deciding to purchase a car. If they do, they frequently communicate with dealerships via phone or online. What impact has this modification had on the experience role within your own team? The fact that consumers now have greater knowledge about a good or service is one significant change for people in sales. However, expertise and knowledge also continue to provide the insight and aptitude needed to make the connections for other professionals. It's true that executives in companies need and want younger generations. However, you also need individuals on your team who have dealt with comparable problems in the past since they can offer important insights into what has previously worked.

Why are experiences and relationships important in marketing and sales?
Clients want to feel understood and heard. Customers desire a company's goods and services to suit their requirements and lifestyles. Additionally, they want the business to support them in the future for any purchases or service needs. Naturally, all of this is financially costly, which is why businesses need to make sure their clients keep purchasing from them. Most businesses, as is well known, spend money on sales and marketing. Both responsibilities

strengthen client relationships and provide clients with a business experience that persuades them to purchase your goods. However, you also need a team with the know-how to use your business information output to inform strategic decisions that are relevant. Put another way, creating reports is insufficient. To make judgments, you need people with business acumen, and that requires experience.

Why does experience matter in business today?

The most successful executives are aware that relationships are key. However, the bond that keeps these connections together is experience. Experience fosters confidence between your business and its clients and enables it to fulfill promises made to them. It also aids in placing the right individuals in the proper positions for your business.

Yes, you should attract tech-savvy individuals. However, you also want individuals who possess critical soft skills related to emotional intelligence. The truth is that having employees that are unable to comprehend technical details and subtleties in addition to other individuals will prevent your firm from succeeding.

Fosters the dedication required to establish a profitable company

If you have a lot of experience starting a business, you are probably doing so because you have observed the problems others in that industry used to face and believe you can solve those problems in a way that would benefit your company. Due to your prior company experience, you will find greater motivation to deliver the ideal solution. However, you might not be as passionate about finding a solution as someone who has been there before and is aware of the problems others are having if your company is merely the result of an internet concept.

provides a market advantage over competitors

There is currently intense competition in every industry more than before. You will need experience-derived knowledge and insight if you want to have any chance. That is the only way you can assist your business in overcoming the formidable competition. Entrepreneurs with extensive experience have a deep understanding of their industry. In this manner, they are conversant with the evolving trends and needs of their clientele. They are able to develop the ideal solution that appeals to their target audience thanks to this expertise. You must understand how to apply your experience if you want to produce a product that appeals to consumers in your business.

Chapter 5

Ignorance: Is It Ever Your Friend?

At work, we communicate with others all the time. Many of these have an effect on our capacity for success. In the event that one of those individuals is unable to fulfill their obligations, what would you do? You will frequently encounter stupidity at work, whether it comes from a coworker or, worse yet, your supervisor. How do you professionally deal with other people's ignorance? How do you choose which battles to enter? How do you guarantee your success in the face of ignorance on the part of others? How can you avoid having your reputation damaged by people believing you don't know enough about your colleagues?

Ignorance and Diversity

I frequently discuss the importance of diversity in the workplace. It might surprise you to learn that even in terms of IQ and common sense, I'm an advocate for diversity. I'm sure it appears counterintuitive. Consider it in this manner. Not every person in the room has to be the most knowledgeable on every subject. Having everyone think they are the most intelligent and educated person participating in every situation would be highly counterproductive. Businesses require a wide range of knowledge, abilities, and insight. A bookish coworker may not always be able to respond quickly and nimbly in professional settings. Occasionally, the astute and streetwise co worker lacks the creativity to generate the big idea. Sometimes the team member with the least amount of talent has an extremely brilliant idea since they don't know how things should" be done in the commercial world. Most businesses find success in finding the proper combination and striking the right balance.

Managing Ignorance.

Notwithstanding the importance of diversity, let me state unequivocally that ignorance of proper workplace conduct is intolerable. Nobody likes to deal with inexperience or ineptitude, especially when success depends on others. Unfortunately, it occurs every day. In many circumstances, businesses tolerate ignorance far longer than they should, even in the face of evidence of detrimental effects. Because of this, your ability to succeed in the workplace depends on your ability to deal with, overcome, and get past ignorance.

These are some strategies that I have found to be effective..

Recognize your weak points .

When you find yourself getting angry at someone you work with frequently for what you believe to be ignorance, stop and look at the bigger picture. We frequently only engage with people in one capacity. That person may interact with others in several capacities. Despite your perception to the contrary, it's possible that someone isn't wholly inadequate in their role. It's possible that you were fortunate enough to have encountered their biggest vulnerability. You may typically make adjustments to the way you manage your relationship with your colleague if you are able to recognize areas of strength (or less weakness) in addition to understanding regions of weakness. Try to limit the amount of their weakness that can affect you. Assign them additional responsibilities within the team in areas that affect people if they excel at numbers but struggle with people. If they excel in interpersonal interactions but struggle with attention to detail, find ways to highlight their strengths while you take care of the minutiae. To eliminate ignorance from the equation, work out an alternative exchange. This is about giving a colleague air cover in their area of weakness and using their strengths to your advantage. By doing this, you safeguard your performance as well. Don't worry about what is good or wrong, fair or unfair. That's just how business works. If not for your coworker, then do it for yourself.

Adjust Your Goals.

Over the course of my career, I've had the incredible fortune to collaborate with some truly talented people. Several of my former coworkers have incredibly distinctions. the first residential high-speed cable

modem company, the original Intel chip, the president

and founder of MTV, the woman of the year in the

telecom sector, the creator of a well-known instant

messaging service, a New York Times best-selling

author, numerous millionaires, and multiple MENSA

members. I consider myself extremely fortunate to

have gained so much knowledge and inspiration from

these people.
Working with talented individuals, however, has the drawback of ruining you. When you work with people who are not only devoid of profound skill of any type, but also uninformed of commercial things, it becomes even more apparent. If you've had the good fortune to be motivated by coworkers, you understand precisely what I mean. Others find it quite challenging to live up to your high standards. Resetting your expectations to a more acceptable level is sometimes all that is necessary. It's possible that your coworkers are not as intelligent as you would want. They might make bad decisions that affect other people by making decisions that don't make sense. You can think to yourself, "They just don't get it."
  However, if you let go of assumptions about what other people ought to be like and accept them for who they are, you

probably will be more tolerant of others'
shortcomings and be able to come up
with inventive solutions to deal with
them.

Always, always, always mitigate.

Whether we like it or not, how we
perform affects how other people
perceive us. Because of this, we need to
exercise caution while letting ignorance
run amok in the workplace. It is only
happiness for those who are ignorant.

Dispute privately.

In every argument, the more intelligent
individual is probably going to get
frustrated first. When we are angry,
especially in front of an audience, we
don't negotiate well. When confronting
an ignorant idea, deed, or behavior,
attempt to do so in private if at all
possible. One way to start these
conversations is by saying, "I'm

frustrated because of." This is the reason I want us to think about it. I'd really like to visit concur. Let's discuss our choices and I will try to comprehend your decision.

Choose your battles wisely.
Occasionally, ignorance doesn't really hurt that much. It is best to let ignorance go, like water off a duck's back, when it is a minor irritation. Draw anything on the paper in front of you, look away, or inhale deeply. Give it up. However, when the stakes are great, ignorance can have a big effect. In some situations, you have to decide which side to support, try your best to negotiate a better result, or escalate the matter to a higher authority.

 As with the previous advice I've given you, focus on the facts and talk about the ramifications. Feelings should be left at the door, and comments of ignorance should only be spoken in your head. Not an exemption.

Put in some effort.
You will occasionally have to accept unfavorable results.
What you may perceive as blatantly stupid may not be so evident to others. Just let the games start and don't become too attached. Try your hardest to contain the damage for the benefit of the company, your clients, your teammates, and yourself. It's simple to just hand the repercussions off to someone else, especially the one who allowed stupidity to enter the room. Avoid doing it. Long-term, it doesn't benefit you very much. Put in some effort.

You never know when it could come in handy.
Being ignorant of widely held notions can help you stay ahead of the crowd. It resembles an artist creating a work of art on a blank canvas. On occasion, it's preferable to start fresh and forge your

own path without letting outside influences contaminate your thoughts. Understanding is vital. Occasionally, however, our capacity to act and form wise decisions is hampered by what we know—or believe we know. We stop being able to innovate because we get wedded to accepted norms. Instead of thinking for ourselves, we blindly follow the crowd. You never know when it could come in handy.

 Being ignorant of widely held notions can help you stay ahead of the crowd. It resembles an artist starting with a blank canvas and creating a masterpiece. On occasion, it's preferable to start fresh and forge your own path without letting outside influences contaminate your thoughts. Understanding is vital. Occasionally, however, our capacity to act and form wise decisions is hampered by what we know—or believe we know. We stop being able to innovate because we get wedded to accepted norms. Instead of thinking for ourselves, we blindly follow the crowd.

"All you need in this life is ignorance and confidence, and then success is sure," is a remark attributed to Mark Twain. Is it possible to dislike this quote? "Success is certain in this life if you can handle ignorance with confidence," is how I would phrase it. To achieve great success, you don't need to be the smartest person in the room. You just need to make sure that you don't fall victim to the room's most uneducated person.

Recognize your areas of weakness, lower your standards, lessen the influence of ignorance around you, and use your judgment to advance your abilities. Relieve yourself as necessary, and use extra creativity to "up" your ignorance. Success is guaranteed only then.

Conclusion

How Large Things Get Completed explores why some concepts, items, and behaviors proliferate like diseases and what we can do to intentionally start and stop such epidemics.